Rising

from
the Rubble

To all government and non-government organisations, emergency services (police, fire and ambulance) and, of course, the many thousands of workers in the Canterbury health system who were involved in the response to, and recovery from, the earthquakes of 2010 and 2011.

Rising

from the Rubble

A health system's extraordinary
response to the Canterbury
earthquakes

Michael Ardagh

Joanne Deely

CANTERBURY UNIVERSITY PRESS

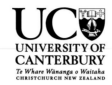

First published in 2018 by
CANTERBURY UNIVERSITY PRESS
University of Canterbury
Private Bag 4800, Christchurch
NEW ZEALAND
www.canterbury.ac.nz/engage/cup

ISBN 978-1-98-850306-6

A catalogue record for this book is available from the
National Library of New Zealand.

Cover and book design and layout: Smartwork Creative, www.smartworkcreative.co.nz

Printed in China through Asia Pacific Offset

Published with assistance from the Canterbury District Health Board
and the Emergency Care Foundation

Contents

Foreword

The Christchurch series of earthquakes put the largest city in New Zealand's South Island under extraordinary pressure. The immediate tragedy of the 22 February quake ripped the heart out of the city in 2011. It destroyed much of its horizontal infrastructure and damaged or destroyed homes, particularly in the eastern part of the city. In modern times at least, it was our most tragic loss of life in a natural disaster. But the event also showed the extraordinary bravery and prompt reaction on the part of the first responders. Thereafter, many continued to show courage and resilience in the face of disaster and acute uncertainty. It is easy to forget that there were months of sleep-ruining quakes prior to and after the 22 February 2011 event, including damaging quakes in September 2010 and June 2011, interspersed with hundreds of frightening aftershocks. This truly put people on edge. This natural disaster was not a finite, singular event like a hurricane, and with its chronic stresses, Christchurch had characteristics more like those of a war zone.

The seismology and geology intrigued seismologists from around the globe. With the possible exception of Japan, it is not often that a major quake and aftershocks occur in such a heavily populated area in a developed economy replete with research-intensive capacities. Thus it soon became one of the most studied seismic events in history. The complex seismology of the earthquake cluster has led to numerous commentaries and scientific papers.

Notwithstanding the immediate rescue and response phase, it is important to understand that any disaster is not over until recovery is complete. The magnitude of the physical damage and associated logistical realities mean that Christchurch is still a long way from full physical repair. As I wrote in my 2011 report to the government after the 22 February quake, the most important aspect of recovery is not the physical rebuild, but the psychology of the people. It can take a long time for them to regain a sense of being in control of their lives and destinies; this includes dealing with the often corrosive effects of financial and insurance worries.

This book is very much about the vitally important emotional recovery of Christchurch's people. In any major disaster, medical attention plays a critical role in the immediate response. When the quake struck, the health care infrastructure itself was seriously damaged and as a result health care workers were under additional severe pressure. These people had their own personal situations and emotions to deal with while working extraordinarily hard, confronting the harrowing human impacts of disaster. Such pressure also applied to the administrators who found themselves confronting decisions beyond those that they had practised for; no disaster plays out in the way that preparatory exercises anticipate. Much has been learnt, both in Christchuch and in Wellington, from these experiences.

This book tells the stories, often in deeply personal ways, about how the health care system and the community staggered and responded. It discusses how the changing circumstances were dealt with while everyone was still discovering the vast extent of the damage that had occurred. Inevitably there were tensions as the country struggled with one of its largest cities under seismic siege while facing enormous logistical challenges and financial responsibilities. Many agencies responded well, but issues did emerge and some of these are discussed in this book. We must learn from these because we will inevitably face another major natural disaster at some time in the future.

My 2011 report advised government on the likely long-term impacts on mental health and how these would become accentuated by fear of further earthquakes and by debates over the rebuild. As a consequence of the earthquakes, there have been changes in how the city operates as the centre has emptied out – it is not clear whether these will entirely return to pre-quake arrangements. There remains huge disruption to roading and an ongoing presence of heavy machinery, while the city's symbolic centre is still in ruins. The reality is that the emotional pressures on the residents of Christchurch will leave scars on the psyche of many people for years. These scars may be subtle, but they are there.

Outside a rather limited and specialist literature, too little is known about the long-term consequences of disaster on individuals and their mental health and about how health care systems and policy systems have to adapt and perform. This is an honest book; emotion and anecdote abound. But underneath it all one senses the presence of strong social determination and a resilient health system that did not just bounce back, but learned along the way.

The last seven years have been a hard, but hopefully an encouraging, journey for Christchurch's health care system, both formal and informal. Michael Ardagh and Joanne Deely's book is a tribute to all and a salutory reminder that the echoes of this tragedy are still resonating for many people. *Rising from the Rubble* will be an invaluable resource for health workers, disaster specialists and policy makers in New Zealand and overseas, and provides an enduring record for all fellow citizens of an important aspect of this extraordinarily challenging time in our history.

Sir Peter Gluckman
Chief Science Advisor to the Prime Minister 2009–2018
August 2018

Preface

As the dust settled after the 22 February 2011 Christchurch earthquake, a cohort of colleagues from the University of Otago, Christchurch, and Canterbury District Health Board (DHB), including ourselves – an emergency medicine specialist, and a health scientist and writer – came together with others to form the Researching the Health Implications of Seismic Events group. The group is often referred to as RHISE, an acronym taken from its full name but which, of course, has connotations with the concept of rising up after being knocked down – a fitting and strongly felt sentiment.

The RHISE group has a number of purposes, with its founding members each conducting their own research. Significantly, the group provides a mechanism for researchers interested in health and the effects of the Canterbury earthquakes on individuals and communities to collaborate on projects and to share their research findings in various forums. Much of the research tells the stories and experiences of those who survived the earthquakes – both the casualties and those who cared for them. A strong motivation for this work is the belief that those who lived and suffered through the Canterbury earthquakes should have their stories told. Indeed, to not do so would be a disrespectful failure to record and acknowledge what they endured, and, furthermore, would be a lost opportunity to inform others who may confront similar events in the future.

The nature of this work means it tends to be published in academic journals held in libraries (both physical and online) that are generally not accessible to the general public. We realised these stories should be told in a way and in a format that everyone can access. We were familiar with the many books published for the public about such topics as everyday heroes rescuing people from the rubble and how people and animals were affected by the 2011 Christchurch earthquake. But we noted a significant dearth of information – an absence of books, columns in newspapers and discussion in other media – about the enormous role played by people involved in health care during and after this event. Furthermore, a comprehensive internet search revealed almost no public literature on health system responses internationally to any prior disasters.

Consequently, it became our primary motivation to write a book that would give the public an understanding of the colossal undertaking that was the health response to the Canterbury earthquakes. We wanted the book to be not only a public record of the Canterbury health system's response, but a celebration of it. It is our view that the health response was remarkably good, and that perhaps the omnipresent, publicly funded, New Zealand health system sometimes is taken for granted and not celebrated enough. The concept for the book was shared with the executive team at Canterbury DHB, and, in 2015, they agreed to provide the requisite support for us to undertake the research, development and writing for the book.

This book contains the definitive history of the Canterbury health system's response to, and recovery from, the February 2011 earthquake, during the initial five years. Today, Canterbury DHB has a world-renowned, well-integrated and patient-centred health system, the result of a process of transformational change that commenced in 2007 to meet the increasing demand for health care. At the time of the earthquake, the Canterbury health system had taken significant steps along that pathway of change. Indeed, the health system's ability to respond to the 2011 earthquake was a direct result of that process.

Beyond the initial response to the earthquake, however, the Canterbury health system needed to resurrect essential services and recover full function. This has been challenging, particularly as the people required to deliver health care were (and some still are) themselves casualties of the earthquake. Many had loved ones, friends or colleagues who were killed or injured, and all were battling the disruption caused by the loss of infrastructure, the prolonged and frustrating challenges of repairing or rebuilding their homes, the heartbreaking damage to the identity of their city, and the disruption to their communities. Remaining strong has come at a cost to many. During the subsequent five years, health care workers and Christchurch's population in general have become fragile. This long and difficult recovery after a major disaster is recognised in some academic circles but it is poorly appreciated generally. The book describes this struggle in detail, with a number of illustrative examples that are both revealing and inspiring, and which will enlighten all readers and provide useful insights for governments and others who might plan for such events.

A number of key themes thread their way through the book. Woven throughout is the importance of collaboration. Both a mechanism and a consequence of the Canterbury health system's journey of change was the evolution of a collaborative and connected community of health care providers, with the result that strong collegial relationships were already in place at the time of the earthquake. This environment proved to be an essential foundation for an effective health response to that event.

Innovation arising from need is another key theme, and it is clear that a post-earthquake sense of freedom from the usual bureaucratic constraints supported and promoted innovative and novel solutions, particularly in the immediate response to the earthquake. Discussion throughout the book points to that innovation, along with collaboration and good relationships, as strengths within the health response. However, these strengths were not always evident when those in the Canterbury health system were working with their governing body in Wellington. It is apparent that a lived experience and a vicarious appreciation of it from afar can lead to different understandings, and, at times, there was a lack of clarity about the respective roles – was it a Canterbury-led response with assistance and facilitation from Wellington, or was the response being led from Wellington?

A strong and enduring theme is the burden of mental illness that is likely to continue in Canterbury long after the earthquakes. We describe a continuum of mental health, from psychosocial wellbeing to severe mental illness, with everyone somewhere on that continuum. Post-earthquake, the majority of people were situated towards the well end of the mental health continuum, with relatively few at the severe end. However, we argue that the mental health of the whole population has shifted along the continuum such that the mental health of each person on that continuum – which, of course, includes all of those who worked in the health system – is at least a little worse than it was before the earthquakes.

This book comprises 16 chapters. The first two chapters provide the backdrop and establish the context for the discussion of the varied topics in the chapters that follow. The opening chapter presents a chilling description of the moments the earthquakes struck an unsuspecting city, and the immediate aftermath, while Chapter 2 depicts the embryonic development of the integrated Canterbury health system that had been established before the 2011 earthquake, and which provided the firm foundation that ultimately allowed the system to respond as well as it did. In Chapter 3 is a fast-moving, action-packed account of Canterbury DHB's management role in the overarching emergency response by the health system, which included shifting hospital wards of patients across the damaged city. The chapter also touches on bureaucratic frustrations that arose when attempting to address some of the challenges. Chapter 4 describes how Christchurch's damaged main public hospital and emergency department received and cared for the many casualties flooding in from the city's shattered central business district. That theme continues in Chapter 5, which recapitulates our published work on the total casualty population from the Christchurch earthquake. New Zealand is uniquely placed to capture the total numbers injured in such an event, as it has a national, government-funded health system with comprehensive recording of accidents and injuries through the Accident Compensation Corporation. Consequently, this chapter delivers a significant insight into who was most vulnerable.

The catastrophic behind-the-scenes damage to the health system's infrastructure, facilities and services is described in Chapter 6, revealing what was required of engineering and maintenance staff to keep a seamless health service going after the disaster. In a similar vein, Chapter 7 portrays the exceptionally organised health response by, and the recovery of, general practitioners, pharmacies and district nursing within their communities, while Chapter 8 furnishes an account of how the region's clinical diagnostic laboratory testing service survived and was able to respond after two of the three laboratories were destroyed by the earthquake. Chapters 9 and 10 recount the experiences of both patients and carers during the evacuation of hundreds of vulnerable people (particularly, older people and those requiring specialist health care, such as dialysis) from Christchurch after the earthquake, their care while they were away and the repatriation effort to bring them home. Chapter 11 depicts how Canterbury DHB's community and public health division collaborated with other organisations in the city-wide response to prevent outbreak of infectious diseases in a city where many people had no reticulated sewage disposal and no clean water.

The health response by Māori and the response to Māori are described in Chapter 12, and have much to tell us about how important is the integration of a response that addresses the needs and capacities of Indigenous people, and the value of grounded and integrated community responses. Chapters 13, 14 and 15 portray the short-, medium- and long-term combined efforts of mental health care providers to support a psychologically injured population recovering from the disaster. The final chapter, Chapter 16, reflects on the important facets of the health response discussed in the earlier chapters, reviewing their significance with regard to the health and wellbeing of Christchurch's population in forthcoming years.

The content of this book came from a variety of sources, including published material in academic and general literature, the authors' personal knowledge of the Canterbury health system and their own experiences during the earthquakes. However, interviews conducted with many who lived and worked through this momentous time were the main source of content. Getting to know these people, listening to their personal stories and gaining their particular insights have been incredible experiences for both of us, and a privilege for which we are very grateful. We provide a list of key contributors, and we acknowledge and thank all of the many people who shared their stories or contributed in numerous and various other ways to this book.

As a consequence of those interviews, this book is able to offer the reader a view of the health system that is uniquely insightful and often deeply personal.

The chapters that follow include both general and more specific insights into aspects of the Canterbury earthquake story. These perspectives are wide-ranging, but they cannot be considered complete as there are innumerable stories from the many thousands of people who provided and received health care in Canterbury during that time.

We acknowledge that some worthy aspects of the health system's response might not have been included and that some important names might not have been mentioned – as an example, the excellent response by the St John ambulance service has not been covered. However, we would suggest that the content of the book has evolved sufficiently during its development to be coherent and adequately comprehensive. Apologies are offered to any who might have been excluded in this pursuit. We also must acknowledge that the perspectives of those who were actively involved with the disaster and the subsequent challenges will likely differ from the perspectives of others who, for example, might have examined the Canterbury health system dispassionately from afar.

This is not a scientific publication and, most certainly, it is not dispassionate. Indeed, the stories that follow are infused with emotions – fear, sadness, anger, pride and, sometimes, joy. It is these, the personal and passionate perspectives of those who lived the experience, which give these interesting stories both volume and importance. It is hoped this book does them justice.

Michael Ardagh and Joanne Deely
Christchurch
May 2018

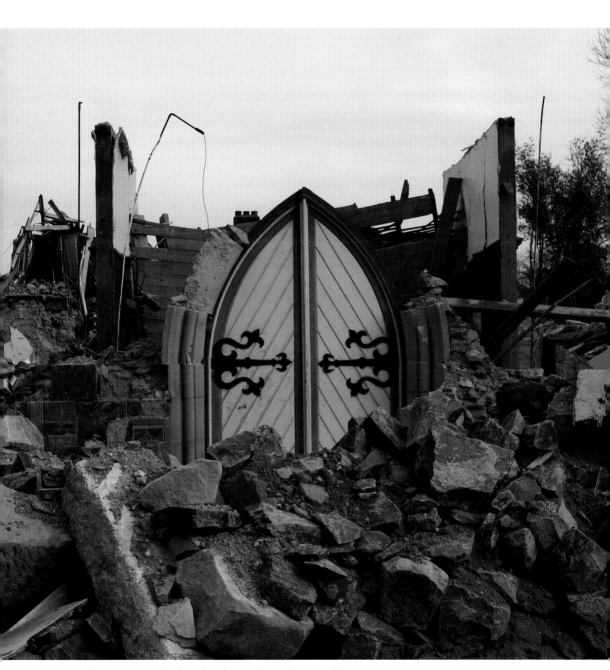

Durham Street Methodist Church, March 2011. (Dave Kelly)

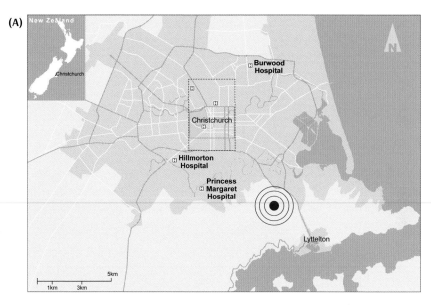

(A)

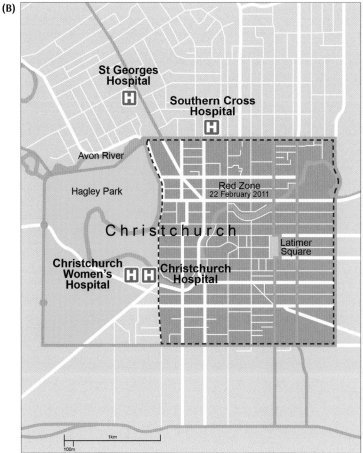

(B)

Map 1 (A) The Christchurch metropolitan area, showing the location of the hospitals (H) and the epicentre of the February 2011 earthquake. The red dashed line approximately shows the boundary of the enlarged map (B) of the Christchurch business district.
(B) The central business district of Christchurch, showing the red zone, the area cordoned-off after the earthquake. (Ardagh, M. et al. (2012). The initial health-system response to the earthquake in Christchurch, New Zealand, in February, 2011. *The Lancet, 379*, 2109–2115, p. 2110)

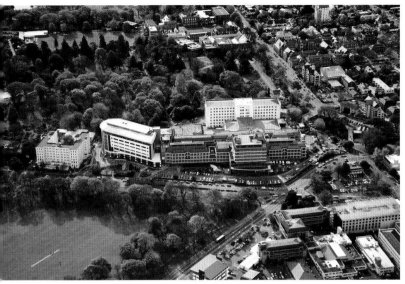

Map 2 Christchurch Hospital and the campus of the University of Otago Christchurch School of Medicine at the intersection of Riccarton Avenue and Hagley Avenue, circa 2012. In the foreground (at right) is the Canterbury Health Laboratories building, and the old nurses' hostel is at far left. (Canterbury DHB)

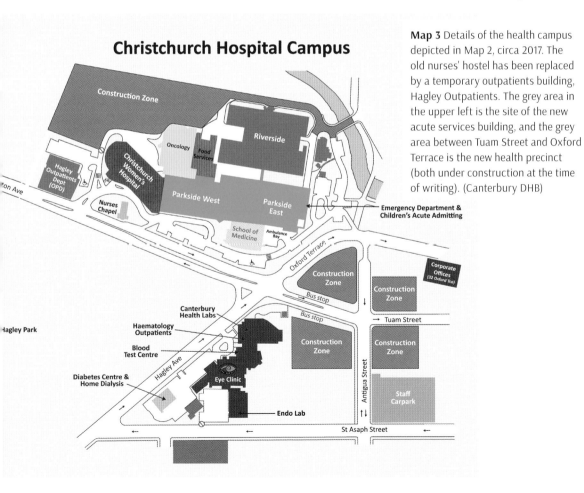

Christchurch Hospital Campus

Construction Zone

Riverside

Oncology
Food Services

Hagley Outpatients Dept (OPD)

Christchurch Women's Hospital

...on Ave

Nurses Chapel

Parkside West

Parkside East

School of Medicine

Ambulance Bay

Emergency Department & Children's Acute Admitting

Oxford Terrace

Construction Zone

Construction Zone

Corporate Offices (32 Oxford Tce)

Canterbury Health Labs

Haematology Outpatients

Blood Test Centre

Bus stop

Bus stop

Tuam Street

Construction Zone

Construction Zone

Hagley Park

Diabetes Centre & Home Dialysis

Hagley Ave

Eye Clinic

Antigua Street

Staff Carpark

Endo Lab

St Asaph Street

Map 3 Details of the health campus depicted in Map 2, circa 2017. The old nurses' hostel has been replaced by a temporary outpatients building, Hagley Outpatients. The grey area in the upper left is the site of the new acute services building, and the grey area between Tuam Street and Oxford Terrace is the new health precinct (both under construction at the time of writing). (Canterbury DHB)

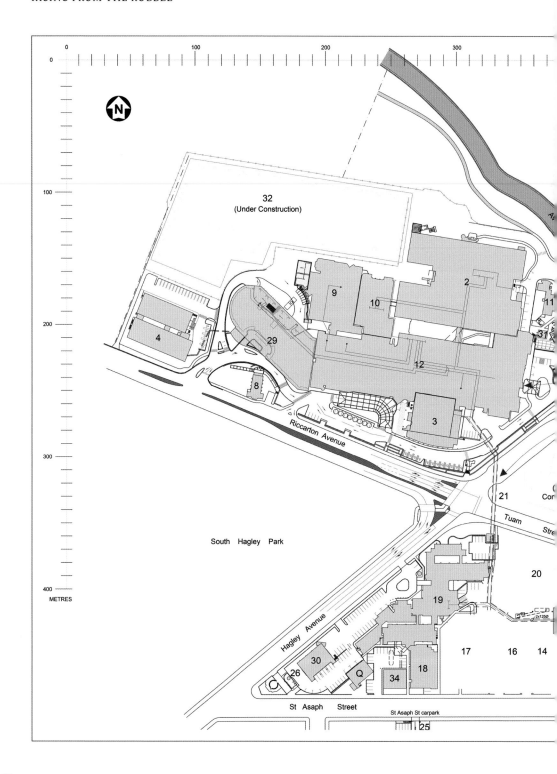

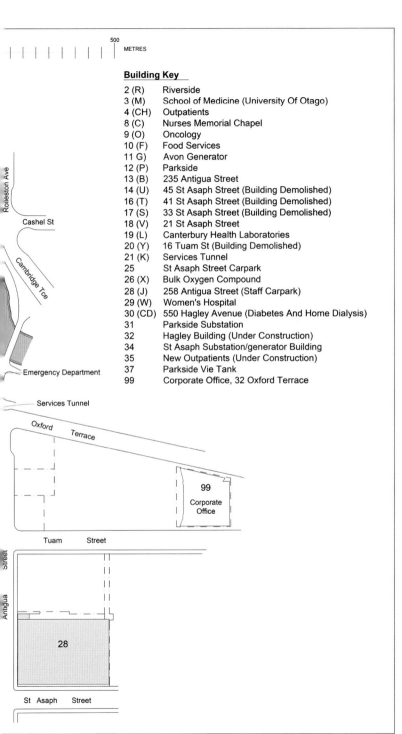

Building Key

2 (R)	Riverside
3 (M)	School of Medicine (University Of Otago)
4 (CH)	Outpatients
8 (C)	Nurses Memorial Chapel
9 (O)	Oncology
10 (F)	Food Services
11 G)	Avon Generator
12 (P)	Parkside
13 (B)	235 Antigua Street
14 (U)	45 St Asaph Street (Building Demolished)
16 (T)	41 St Asaph Street (Building Demolished)
17 (S)	33 St Asaph Street (Building Demolished)
18 (V)	21 St Asaph Street
19 (L)	Canterbury Health Laboratories
20 (Y)	16 Tuam St (Building Demolished)
21 (K)	Services Tunnel
25	St Asaph Street Carpark
26 (X)	Bulk Oxygen Compound
28 (J)	258 Antigua Street (Staff Carpark)
29 (W)	Women's Hospital
30 (CD)	550 Hagley Avenue (Diabetes And Home Dialysis)
31	Parkside Substation
32	Hagley Building (Under Construction)
34	St Asaph Substation/generator Building
35	New Outpatients (Under Construction)
37	Parkside Vie Tank
99	Corporate Office, 32 Oxford Terrace

Map 4 Map of the Christchurch Hospital campus showing the tunnel linking the energy plant (13) to Canterbury Health Laboratories (19), Christchurch Hospital (2, 12) and Christchurch Women's Hospital (29). (Terry Walker, Canterbury DHB)

Following pages: Victoria Street, March 2011, showing clock stopped at the time of the earthquake. (Dave Kelly)

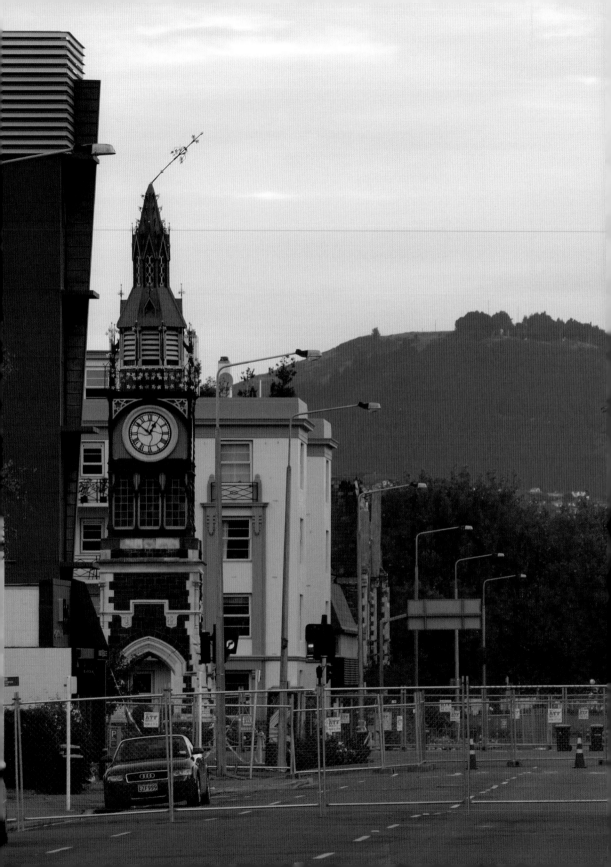

Chapter 1

A TIME AND A PLACE:
12.51PM, 22 FEBRUARY 2011, CHRISTCHURCH CITY, CANTERBURY, NEW ZEALAND

AT 4.35AM ON SATURDAY, 4 SEPTEMBER 2010, an earthquake with a magnitude of 7.1 emanated from an epicentre 40 kilometres west of Christchurch near the town of Darfield on the Canterbury Plains (see Fig. 1.1). It was a shallow earthquake with a depth of only 10 kilometres, and caused a shaking intensity described on the Modified Mercalli Intensity scale[1] as 'extreme'. In Christchurch City damage was significant, with windows broken and many shop façades collapsing to the ground. Brick chimneys were traditionally a common feature of Canterbury homes but some chimneys were so old that the binding mortar was dry and crumbling, leaving the chimneys as little more than a balanced stacks of bricks sitting on roofs. The earthquake caused many chimneys to fall, some collapsing through roofs onto sleeping inhabitants in the rooms below.

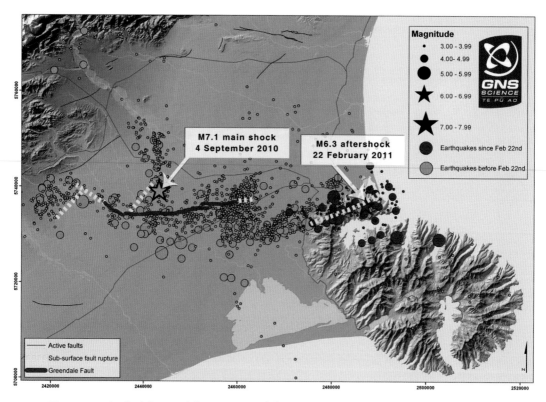

Figure 1.1 Major fault lines and the epicentres of the Canterbury earthquakes of 2010 and 2011. (GNS Science)

The fault movement opened the surface of the earth, twisting and bending previously straight roads and lines of trees (see Fig. 1.2). Many homes and buildings suffered some damage, particularly in the proximate country and towns, and the people became acquainted with the concept of liquefaction – a process whereby the shaking from the earthquake brought a muddy mixture of subterranean silt, fine sand and water through cracks to the surface, often leaving small, volcano-like cones on open ground, and sometimes flooding large areas. Liquefaction mud bubbled up under solid structures – such as roads or floors – lifting and buckling them, and in other areas, liquefaction caused some buildings to sink.

Despite the earthquake's intensity, its epicentre was located in an area of relatively low population density and most people were in bed, meaning no deaths were directly attributable to the earthquake and that most of the approximately 100 injuries were not severe.

Even so, all in the region had been woken – both from their weekend sleep and from their seismic naïvety. As the spring turned to summer and Christmas came and went, many believed that the 'big one' had also come and gone, and that life should go on, albeit with more awareness and better preparation – just in case.

New Zealand, as a small, narrow land mass surrounded by a great deal of ocean, is always subject to variable weather conditions, but in Canterbury the patterns are largely familiar. Almost six months after the September earthquake, Tuesday 22 February 2011 was a warm summer day in Christchurch, with a northwest foehn wind[2] coming down from the mountains to the west of Christchurch and gathering warmth as it crossed the land. Typically, as a circulating weather system travels east from Australia over the Tasman Sea, the prevailing northwesterly flow of air shifts to the southwest, bringing with it colder temperatures and rain. This change in the weather was forecast; however, for the moment, the warm temperatures prevailed and people went out and about the town for lunch.

The time was 12.51pm when the most destructive earthquake struck on 22 February 2011.

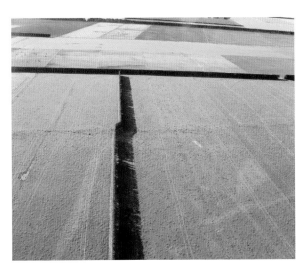

Figure 1.2 Displacement of a line of trees caused by the rupture of the earth's surface along the Greendale Fault on 4 September 2010. Part of the tree line has been offset horizontally by about 3.5 metres. (GNS Science and the GeoNet project. Photographer David Barrell)

Under the hills of the erstwhile volcanic rim adjacent to Christchurch, and just five kilometres deep and within 10 kilometres of the central city, a previously unnamed fault liberated a 6.3 magnitude earthquake. Officially it was an aftershock of the Darfield earthquake in September but it was far more destructive than the main shock. From the epicentre radiated seismic waves. They raced through the soft substrate, fractured hard substrate and bounced rocks about. The waves of energy that struck Christchurch's city centre were followed closely by others and then more again as they reflected off the volcanic rock of the Port Hills towards the city.

Into that mild, sunny, unsuspecting lunchtime in the city streets came a rumbling crescendo, like an approaching truck, soon followed by the shaking. The movement of the ground was violent for all, but people described it differently, depending on where they were and what they were doing. For many, the shaking started with violent jerks, lifting and crashing, lifting and crashing, again and again, until the jerks became waves and, finally, only ripples were left. Few people could stand and those who did strained their

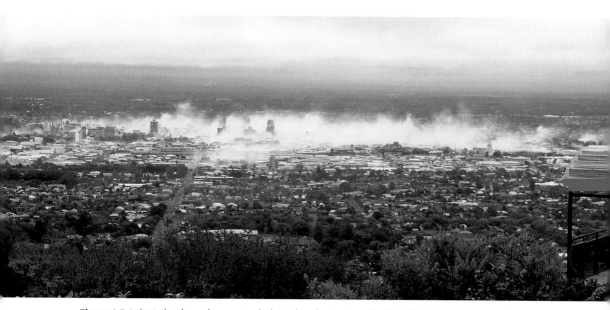

Figure 1.3 A dust cloud envelops central Christchurch minutes after the 22 February 2011 earthquake struck. (Gilly Needham)

limbs, muscles and joints to stay upright. Many objects that were unsecured became projectiles and the masonry fronts of the city shops and buildings tumbled like avalanches of rubble onto the streets below, crushing cars, buses and pedestrians. Some people who could secure sufficient footing to run outside, seeking safety, were instead greeted by this hazard.

Roads cracked and buckled, and bridges broke and twisted. Liquefied mud and silt bubbled up from the depths, warping the surface where it could not break through. In suburbs to the east of the city, where the land was softer and the water table higher, silt flooded streets and houses, and sinkholes formed, claiming the odd passing car (see Fig. 1.4). Hagley Park, the central park of Christchurch, was pock-marked with thousands of small, liquefaction 'volcanoes'. It is estimated that 400 000 tonnes of silt made its way to the surface, where much of it subsequently dried and blew about in the warm summer winds of the following weeks (possibly contributing to a perceptibly high incidence of respiratory diseases in post-earthquake Christchurch).

City buildings were damaged, although people were able to evacuate most of them – albeit down damaged stairwells or fire escapes, or even by abseiling down walls after climbing out of damaged windows. In a city where the high structural integrity of the buildings undoubtedly protected many who might otherwise have perished, thereby preventing greater loss of life, two buildings failed catastrophically. The Canterbury Television (CTV) building collapsed, leaving only its burning lift-shaft standing tall among six storeys of pancaked

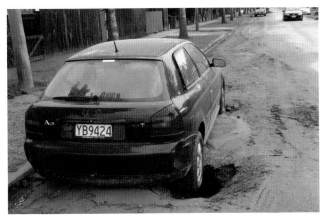

Figure 1.4 Sinkhole and liquefaction in Oxley Avenue, February 2011. (Dave Kelly)

concrete. In that collapsed building, 115 lives were lost, including many international students at an English language school and staff of a medical clinic. A subsequent government review found the construction of this particular building to be sadly wanting. The Pyne Gould Corporation (PGC) building, a four-storey building of reinforced concrete built in the early 1960s, also collapsed, taking 18 lives. Of the 185 deaths officially attributed to the earthquake of 22 February 2011, these two buildings contributed 133. However, death and injury occurred throughout the city, and damage was widespread.

Tens of thousands of houses needed demolition, and large areas of previously inhabited suburbs were 'red-zoned' – that is, the land was defined as being inappropriate for re-building houses. The eastern suburbs of Christchurch were particularly hard hit, experiencing extensive damage from liquefaction. The effect was to compound the pre-existing socioeconomic deprivation evident in that part of the city to produce a much worse disaster impact for this population. The loss of electricity, and limited or no access to clean drinking water or sewage disposal, were widespread, but inevitably affected the eastern suburbs more severely and for longer compared with other areas of Christchurch.

However, no citizen of Christchurch was immune to the effects of this earthquake. Within hours, 182 people were dead, and the earthquake would claim three more lives over the ensuing days. The death toll might be counted higher if some of the deaths of the frail and elderly were attributed to it; if some of the subsequent deaths on the damaged roads were counted; or if some of the deaths from heart attacks were included. Many heart attacks probably were precipitated by earthquake-related stress. In addition, many thousands of people were injured, with a significant number requiring hospital treatment.

A great many Christchurch people were displaced, forced to live in temporary or makeshift accommodation, and every citizen can talk of the innovations necessary for washing and toileting in post-earthquake Christchurch. Indeed, the stories of temporary toilets in back yards and gardens have been the subject of much discussion in both the mainstream and social media.

No matter how this earthquake is viewed, how the hardships are described or the casualties are counted, it was a most destructive event. The movement underfoot was severe. Peak ground accelerations – a measure of the violence of the movement of the earth – were up to 2.2 times the acceleration due to gravity (2.2G), the highest vertical peak ground accelerations ever recorded. Although extremely violent, this earthquake was brief, lasting only about 10 seconds in duration. However, it was just one shock (albeit the most destructive) in a long and continuing sequence of earthquakes. Many thousands of aftershocks continued for months after the initial event, with many measuring above magnitude 4 on the Richter scale and a number measuring a damaging magnitude 5, a factor of 10 greater.

There is a story about an experiment involving laboratory rats. The rats kept in one cage were subject to electric shocks through the wired-up floor of their cage. The shocks were of consistent voltage and were regularly timed. The rats learned to predict when the shocks would occur, and would eat, drink and thrive between shocks, only to hunker down when they knew a shock was coming. In another cage, other rats were subject to the same total number and voltage of shocks as those in the first cage, but the shocks came randomly and were of varying severity. These rats could not eat or sleep, and withered as a consequence.

The experience of the people of Christchurch after the February 2011 earthquake might be compared to that of the rats in the second cage – unwilling participants in a divine experiment, amid destruction and disruption, with aftershocks striking without warning and each with the potential to be the one that might end it all. In that environment, many services needed to respond, heal, recover and contribute to the recovery of the region. The Canterbury health system was one of those many services, and its story is remarkable. The chapters that follow tell that remarkable story.

Following pages: Christchurch and the Canterbury Plains from the Port Hills, September 2006. (Wikimedia Commons. Photographer: P. Stalder)

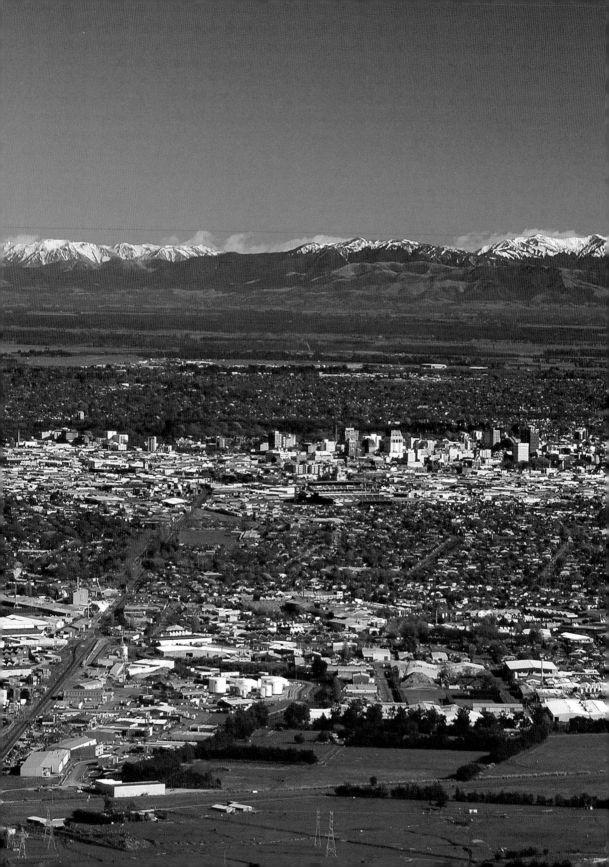